BIGGER ISN'T ALWAYS BETTER

CHOOSING YOUR PORTIONS

OBESITY & KIDS

BIGGER ISN'T ALWAYS BETTER

CHOOSING YOUR PORTIONS

BY RAE SIMONS

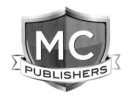

Mason Crest Publishers

MASON CREST PUBLISHERS INC.
370 Reed Road
Broomall, Pennsylvania 19008
(866)MCP-BOOK (toll free)
www.masoncrest.com

First Printing
9 8 7 6 5 4 3 2 1

Library of Congress Cataloging-in-Publication Data

Simons, Rae, 1957–
 Bigger isn't always better : choosing your portions / by Rae Simons.
     p. cm.
 Includes bibliographical references and index.
  ISBN 978-1-4222-1706-1   ISBN 978-1-4222-1705-4 (series)
  ISBN 978-1-4222-1894-5 (pbk.)   ISBN 978-1-4222-1893-8 (pbk series)
 1. Food portions—Juvenile literature. 2. Diet—Juvenile literature. 3. Food habits-Juvenile literature. I. Title.
 RA784.S557 2011
 613.2—dc22
                        2010028159

Design by MK Bassett-Harvey.
Produced by Harding House Publishing Service, Inc.
www.hardinghousepages.com
Cover design by Torque Advertising + Design.
Printed in USA by Bang Printing.

CONTENTS

INTRODUCTION
FOR THE TEACHERS

We as a society often reserve our harshest criticism for those conditions we understand the least. Such is the case for obesity. Obesity is a chronic and often-fatal disease that accounts for 400,000 deaths each year. It is second only to smoking as a cause of premature death in the United States. People suffering from obesity need understanding, support, and medical assistance. Yet what they often receive is scorn.

Today, children are the fastest growing segment of the obese population in the United States. This constitutes a public health crisis of enormous proportions. Living with childhood obesity affects self-esteem, which down the road can affect employment and attainment of higher education. But childhood obesity is much more than a social stigma. It has serious health consequences.

Childhood obesity increases the risk for poor health in adulthood—but also even during childhood. Depression, diabetes, asthma, gallstones, orthopedic diseases, and other obesity-related conditions are all on the rise in children. Recent estimates suggest that 30 to 50 percent of children born in 2000 will develop type 2 diabetes mellitus, a leading cause of preventable blindness, kidney failure, heart disease, stroke, and amputations. Obesity is undoubtedly the most pressing nutritional disorder among young people today.

If we are to reverse obesity's current trend, there must be family, community, and national objectives promoting healthy eating and exercise. As a nation, we must demand broad-based public-health initiatives to limit TV watching, curtail junk food advertising toward children, and promote physical activity. More than rhetoric, these need to be our rallying cry. Anything short of this will eventually fail, and within our lifetime obesity will become the leading cause of death in the United States if not in the world. This series is an excellent first step in battling the obesity crisis by educating young children about the risks, the realities, and what they can do to build healthy lifestyles right now.

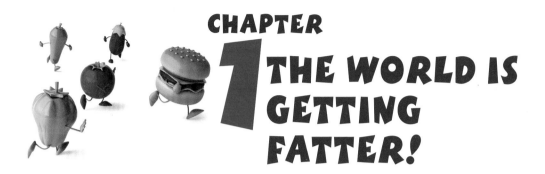

CHAPTER 1
THE WORLD IS GETTING FATTER!

Did you know that people all over the globe are getting fatter? There are more than 1 billion adults around the world who are *overweight*. At least 300 million of them are *obese*.

But it's not just grownups who are overweight and obese. More and more children are overweight too, even very young children. Around the world, at least 42 million children who are younger than five are overweight. In the United States alone, 15 percent of all children between the ages of 6 and 11 are overweight.

That means that if you have 100 children in a room, chances are 15 of them would be overweight.

And if you were to put 100 kids who were between the ages of 12 and 19 all in one room, you'd be likely to find that 18 of them (18 percent) would be overweight.

And then, if you put 100 grownups together, 67 of them would be overweight or obese. That's more than two-thirds of all grownups!

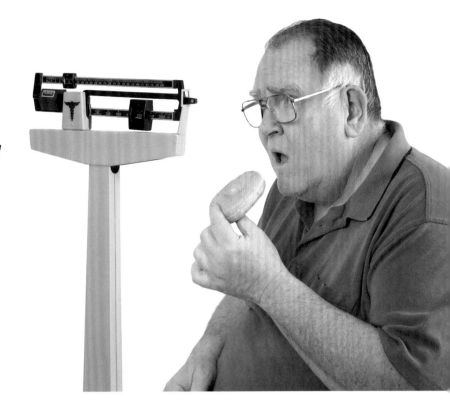

Lots of grownups in the world are overweight. This used to be a problem that mostly just happened in countries like the United States, but as food becomes more available around the world, more people are overweight in other parts of the world as well.

Both **obese** and **overweight** mean a person has too much body fat, so much so that it's a health risk. But a person who is obese has much more fat than a person who is overweight, and the health risks are greater as well.

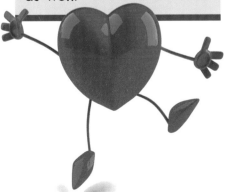

HOW DID WE GET SO FAT?

People weren't always fat. Up until the twentieth century, most people simply worked too hard to be overweight. Maybe a few very wealthy people ate more calories than they used—but around the world, most people were farmers who worked hard to grow their food.

Today's obesity problem started in America, where most people eat more calories than they really need. Over the past fifty years or so, the *lifestyle* of the United States has been spreading all around the world. There are good things about that— and there are bad. America's obese lifestyle is one of the not-so-good things.

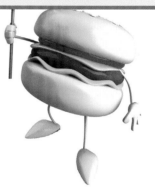

DID YOU KNOW?

Calories are a way to measure what's in the food we eat. We use inches and feet (or centimeters and meters) to measure how long or tall something is; we use pints and quarts (or liters) to measure liquids like milk and soda—and we use calories to measure how much energy is in a certain food.

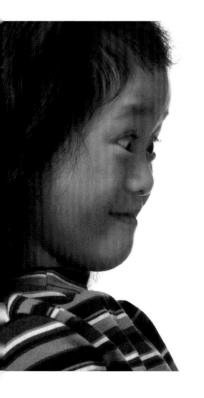

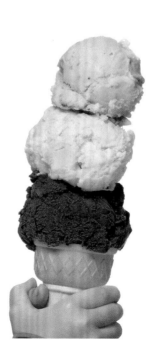

If you're like many people, you crave sweet or fatty foods (like ice cream!). That may be because early humans spent nearly every moment chasing after their food. Once they caught it, they needed to eat as much as they could because there might not be any more tomorrow. Those who ate the most survived—and those who ate the least died. It's not easy to fight evolution!

When the first white settlers came to North America, they had never seen so much farmland. As the years went by, more and more people crossed the Atlantic Ocean. Many of them came because they did not have enough to eat in their old homes in Europe.

America was a big land. The settlers felt as though it were so big that there was bound to be plenty for everyone. BIGNESS became an important part of how Americans thought about themselves and their country.

American farmers began growing acres of wheat and corn. They fed most of the corn to thousands and thousands of cows, chickens, and pigs.

Most of the people of the United States were no longer poor and hungry, the way many of them had once been on their small farms in their small countries back in Europe. Instead, Americans ate hearty meals of beef and potatoes, chicken and dumplings, ham and biscuits. These enormous meals were a part of being an American.

THE BIGGER THE BETTER

Americans started believing that BIG things were better than small things. Big houses were better than small houses, for example. Enormous, gas-guzzling cars were better than small, *compact* cars. While other countries valued things that took up little space and worked well, Americans wanted things to be big simply for bigness sake!

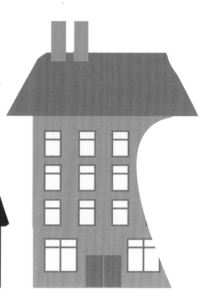

Something that is **compact** doesn't take up much room. It fits everything into a small space.

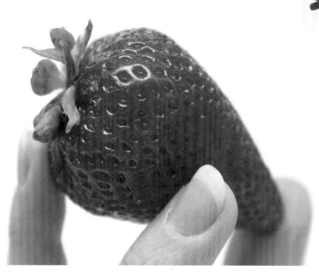

The demand for big strawberries led to fruit scientists developing giant fruit like that shown here. These enormous strawberries also lasted better while being shipped from the strawberry fields of California to the rest of the United States—and, because they were so big, they were faster (and cheaper) to pick.

American scientists started developing bigger fruits and vegetables for farmers to grow. These often didn't taste as good as the smaller ones—but they were BIG! Restaurants served larger portions. Baked goods swelled to twice their former size. Even plates and bowls got bigger!

And as everything that Americans did and ate got larger and larger, so did the Americans themselves!

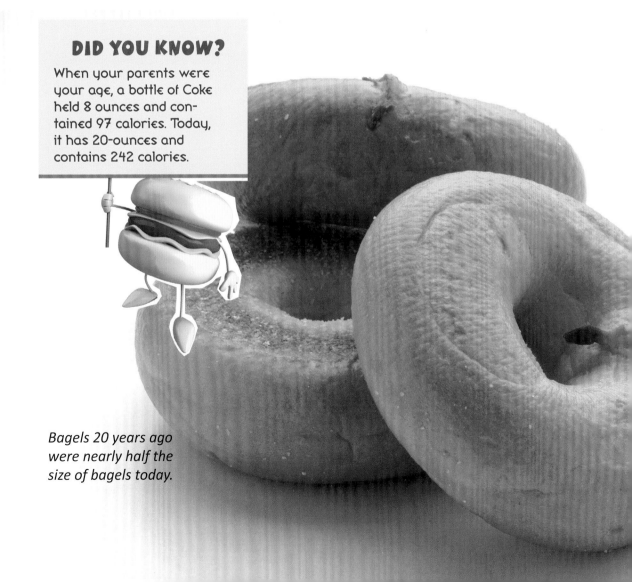

DID YOU KNOW?

When your parents were your age, a bottle of Coke held 8 ounces and contained 97 calories. Today, it has 20-ounces and contains 242 calories.

Bagels 20 years ago were nearly half the size of bagels today.

BEAUTIFUL BIG BODIES

Back in the 1800s, the main things that made people get sick or die were diseases that spread from person to person. Peo-

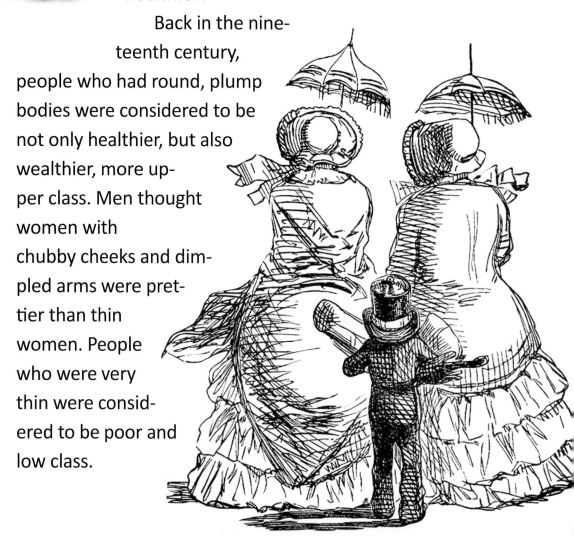

ple were more likely to catch these diseases if they didn't have a healthy diet, so doctors and health officials encouraged people to eat more of all kinds of food. Doctors even told their patients to gain weight in order to be healthier!

Back in the nineteenth century, people who had round, plump bodies were considered to be not only healthier, but also wealthier, more upper class. Men thought women with chubby cheeks and dimpled arms were prettier than thin women. People who were very thin were considered to be poor and low class.

As the 1800s went past, however, the world changed. New machines of all sorts were being invented, and many of these machines helped grow food, package it, and move it from place to place much more cheaply and quickly. This meant that you no longer had to be rich in order to have plenty of food.

By the 1920s, upper-class people considered thinness to be a sign of beauty and wealth. Women who had hollow cheeks and bony hips were now considered to be the prettiest. No one wanted to be fat anymore, and doctors were now advising their patient to lose weight.

But food was plentiful in the United States—and Americans were still gaining weight. So were people in other parts of the world.

Get Thinner

A WORLD THAT SITS

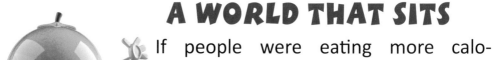

If people were eating more calories but exercising more, the world wouldn't have such a big problem. But instead, they're doing just the opposite—they're eating more and exercising less. This is another part of America's unhealthy lifestyle.

Even fifty years ago, most grownups had plenty of physical work to do that kept them active. Keeping a house clean and growing food took up a lot of time—and it burned a lot of calories. Children had chores to do as well, and when their chores were done, they played games like tag and hide-and-go-seek and hopscotch. All these games involved MOVING. In those days, people moved their bodies every single day.

But that's not the way we live today. Laborsaving inventions like washing machines and vacuum cleaners mean we can keep our homes and clothing clean without working so hard. We buy our food at the grocery store, and often times, it comes in quick, easy-to-fix packages—or we eat out at a restaurant. Daily life just doesn't take as much effort as it once did.

That seems like a good thing. After all, if we have less work to do, then we have more time to enjoy ourselves. And that would be fine too—except the things we do today to enjoy ourselves often don't involve moving our bodies.

Think about what most people do every day. Many grown-ups work in an office where they sit in front of a computer all day. Children go to school, where for much of the day they sit at desks. In the evenings, families come home from school and from work—and then what do they do? Chances are, they sit down and watch television. They might listen to music on their iPods or MP3 players. Or they sit at their computers and play games or surf the Net.

And then they go to bed, get up the next morning—and spend another day sitting. No wonder so many adults and children are obese or overweight!

DID YOU KNOW?

Healthy bodies come in many shapes. Some are small and slender, but others are naturally larger. This doesn't mean they're necessarily overweight!

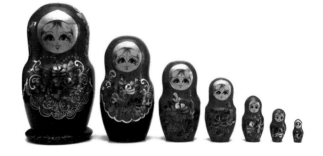

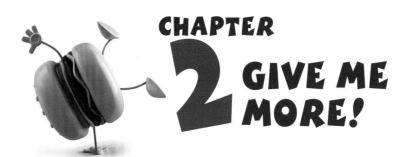

CHAPTER 2 GIVE ME MORE!

CHOOSING THE BIG PIECE

If you had to choose between a big piece of cake and a small piece of cake, which would you choose? What about if someone offered you a one-scoop ice cream cone or a three-scoop cone—which one would you want?

If you're like most people, you'll pick the bigger piece of cake and the larger ice cream cone. It doesn't matter how much we really think we want, or even how hungry we are. We just *assume* that bigger is better.

A hundred years ago, many people in America had to make do with small portions of food. In places of the world where food is *scarce*, people still survive on whatever they have, which may not be very much! Maybe it was times like that, when there wasn't enough food to go around, that made people start feeling as though they had to grab as much food as they could whenever they had the chance.

> **Assume** means you think something's true even though you don't have any proof.
>
> If something is **scarce,** there's not enough of it.

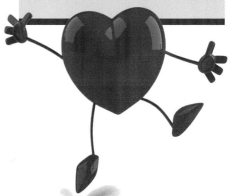

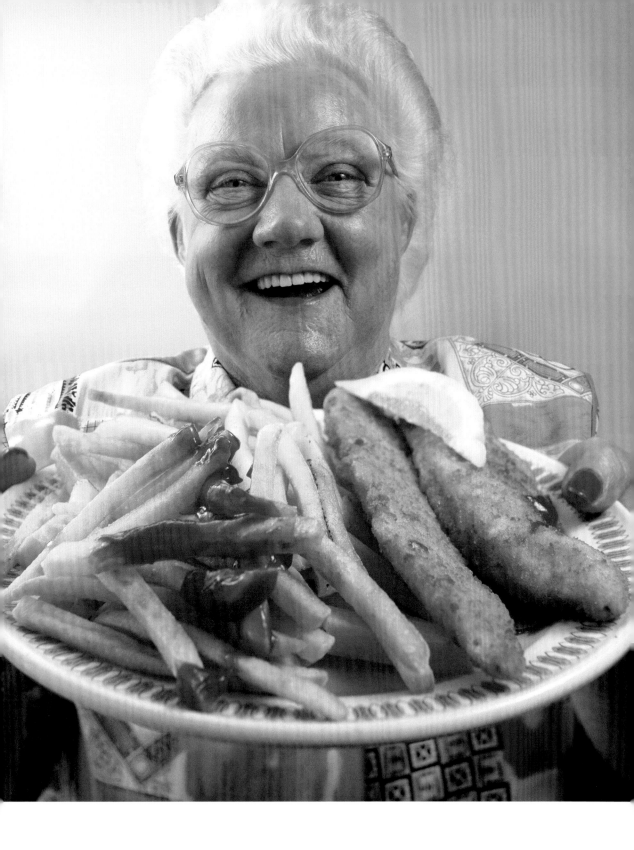

GOOD DEALS

People like a good deal. They like to feel as though they're getting the most for their money.

This attitude goes along with feeling as though bigger is better. If you could find a small car for $15,000 or a big car for the same amount, why wouldn't you want the bigger car? Or if you could buy a big house for the same money as a small house, you'd take the bigger house, right? It seems to make sense. Why would you want to turn down bargains like that?

The problem, though, is that there's an extra price you pay when you choose the bigger thing. Big cars use more gas than small cars, so in the long run, bigger cars cost a lot more to drive. Bigger houses use more electricity and heating fuel than smaller houses, so a big house turns out to be more expensive to own than a small house.

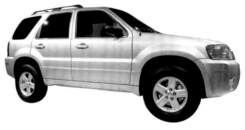

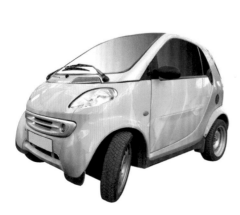

Americans like big things, including big cars. In other parts of the world, however, more people drive smaller cars that use less fuel, like the Smart Car shown here to the left.

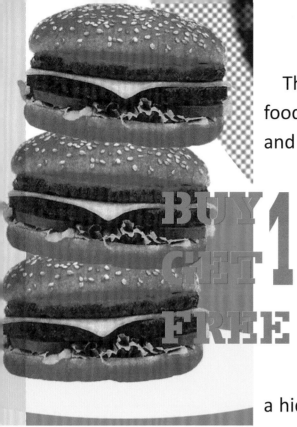

The same is true when it comes to food. If you can buy one hamburger and get another one free, it seems like a great deal. Who would want to turn it down? Or if you can pay the same price for a small bottle of soda as you would for a larger bottle, of course you'd take the bigger bottle. But just like with cars and houses, we end up paying a hidden cost when we choose bigger servings.

If you eat twice as many hamburgers and drink twice as much soda day after day, you're eating more food than your body needs. And that's not good for your body!

Some people think that being overweight doesn't look as nice as being thin, but that's not the real problem. Bodies come in all different shapes and sizes, and you should never think less of someone because of the size of his body. But being overweight causes a lot of health problems. It can make you get sick with serious diseases.

So when you think about it, those great deals on hamburgers and soda aren't such a bargain after all!

PACKAGES AND PORTIONS

Have you ever heard the ***expression***, "Your eyes are bigger than your stomach"? In other words, you want more based on what something looks like rather than the actual space in your stomach.

An **expression** is a figure of speech. It's words people use to express a thought or idea.

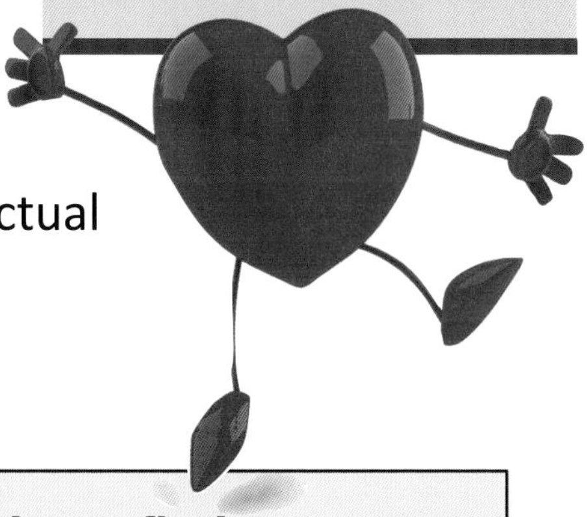

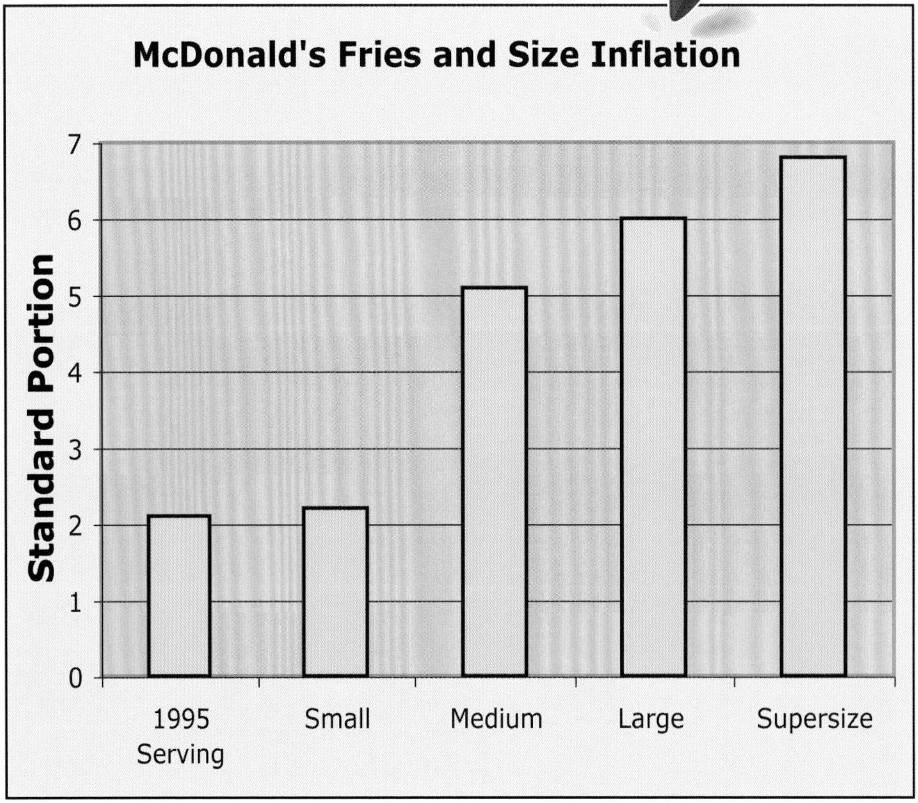
McDonald's Fries and Size Inflation
Standard Portion
0
1
2
3
4
5
6
7
1995 Serving
Small
Medium
Large
Supersize

Fast-food restaurants know the way people's minds work. They know that people like bigger portions. They know that people are more likely to buy more if the serving sizes are bigger. So fast-food restaurants like McDonalds® and Burger King® started making their servings bigger and bigger. French fries, for example, started coming in packages that were larger and larger.

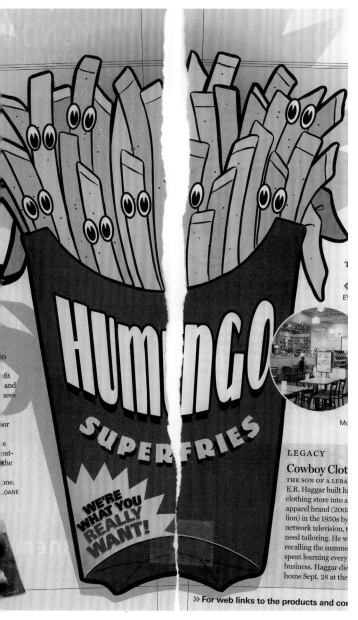

The graph on the opposite page shows the way serving sizes have gotten larger over the years since 1995. Today's "small" is slightly bigger than the "regular" size in 1995—and today's "supersize" is nearly three times as big! If it's big, we think it's better.

But it's not.

PORTION DISTORTION

It's not just fast-food servings that have been getting bigger over the years. Other portion sizes have been getting larger too.

Have you ever ordered spaghetti at a restaurant—and ended up with a bowl of pasta big enough to feed your entire family? Have you ever seen your dad eat a steak the size of a platter at a restaurant?

Lots of other restaurants besides fast-food places now serve enormous portions as well. There's this whole mindset in place that says bigger is always better!

The **USDA** stands for the United States Department of Agriculture. It's the part of the American government that takes care of farming and food.

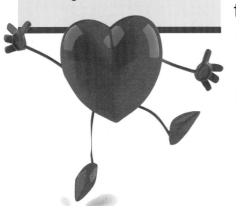

If you look at the graph below, you'll see how much bigger typical-sized restaurant portions are compared to what the *USDA* considers to be a serving. The size of the bagel or steak you get in a restaurant is now actually two servings worth. The average restaurant muffin is more than three times what is considered to be a serving. Dishes of pasta almost equal five servings. (See, they really COULD feed your whole family!) And "home-baked" restaurant cookies are nearly seven times what would be an ordinary serving!

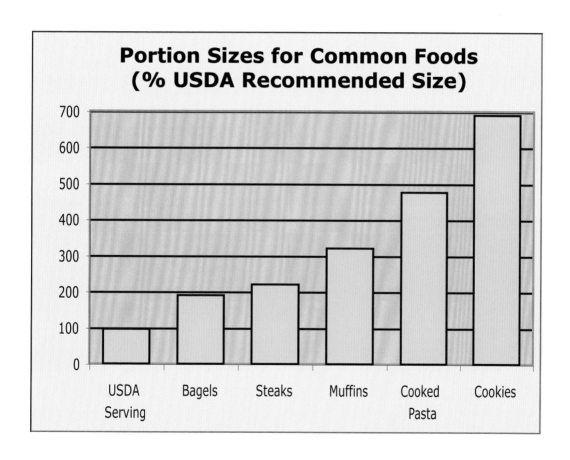

PORTION SIZES AND WAIST SIZES

A group of doctors studied five kinds of food—hamburgers, Mexican food, soft drinks, snacks, and pizza—and found that serving sizes for all of them except pizza had gotten bigger since 1971. Hamburgers today are one-fifth bigger than they were in 1971. A plate of Mexican food is usually one-quarter bigger. In 1971, most soft drinks were 12 ounces, but today,

WORLDWIDE WAISTLINES				
Rank	Country	Age	Gender	Percentage Overweight
1	United States	13	Girls	10.80
2	Portugal	13	Girls	8.30
3	Ireland	13	Girls	6.60
15	Lithuania	13	Girls	2.60
1	United States	15	Girls	15.10
2	Portugal	15	Girls	7.00
3	Denmark	15	Girls	6.50
15	Lithuania	15	Girls	2.10
1	United States	13	Boys	12.6
2	Greece	13	Boys	8.9
3	Ireland	13	Boys	7.0
15	Lithuania	13	Boys	1.8
1	United States	15	Boys	13.9
2	Greece	15	Boys	10.8
3	Israel	15	Boys	6.8
15	Lithuania	15	Boys	.08

many are 20 ounces—and they come with free refills. And serving sizes for snack foods like potato chips and pretzels are two-thirds bigger than they once were! The doctors also discovered that it's not just at restaurants where serving sizes are bigger. People are eating bigger servings at home too.

Serving sizes are connected to our waist sizes. That just makes sense. The graph on the page to the left shows the three countries that rank the highest for having the largest percentages of overweight thirteen-year-old girls—the United States, Portugal, and Ireland. These three countries also have some of the largest portion sizes in the world. Meanwhile, Lithuania has a very small percentage of overweight girls—and their portion sizes are smaller too.

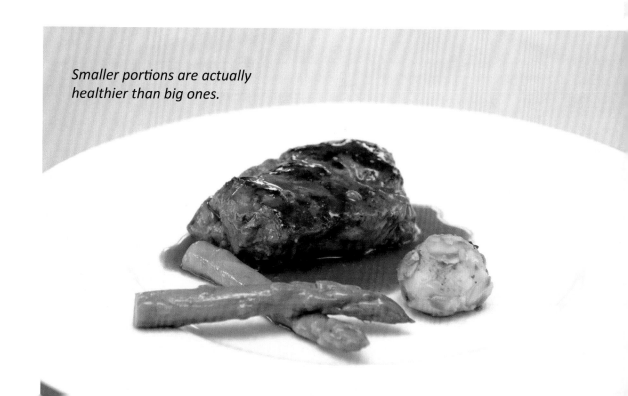

Smaller portions are actually healthier than big ones.

MORE FOOD MEANS MORE CALORIES

Of course, just because you're given a lot of food, doesn't mean you have to eat it all. But chances are you will! Even if you don't eat the whole thing, you'll at least eat more than you would have if you'd been given a smaller serving.

Another group of doctors proved that this was true. They gave people two meals on two different days. Each meal was macaroni and cheese, but one time the doctors gave the people small servings and the other time they gave them big servings. Both times, the doctors told the people to eat until they were full.

Not all of the people cleaned their plates either time (even when the servings were small)—but even if they didn't finish all the food they'd been given, they all ate about a third more when they had big servings than when they had small servings.

You know what else? The people told the doctors they hadn't even noticed that the servings were different sizes!

A Meal at McDonald's

Menu Item	Calories	Fat Grams	Protein Grams	Carbs, Grams
Big Mac™	560	32.4	25.2	43
Fries, large	400	21.6	5.6	46
Shake, chocolate	320	1.7	11.6	66
TOTALS	1280	55.5	42.4	155

Source: McDonald's and USDA data bases

The real problem with people eating servings that are so much bigger than they once were is calories. Look at the chart at the top of the page. You'll see that if you eat a "normal" meal at MacDonalds—a Big Mac®, fries, and a milkshake—you're consuming 1,280 calories. This is nearly two-thirds of the number of calories the average woman should eat in a day, and about half of what the average man should eat. If you eat a child's meal, it's not so bad, of course, in terms of calories. The average Happy Meal® at MacDonalds is about 600 calories, which is the right number for a child's meal. The problem here, though, is whether your body is getting the things it needs along with those calories.

CHAPTER 3

WHAT DO WE REALLY NEED TO BE HEALTHY?

Scientists have discovered the best combination of foods your body needs to be healthy. A diagram of this combination looks like a pyramid, with the foods you need to eat more at the bottom, and the foods you need to eat less at the top. The USDA has created a picture called "MyPyramid" (shown on the opposite page) to help you understand better how much and what kinds of foods you need to eat.

The different colors in the pyramid represent different kinds of food you need to eat each day—grains, vegetables, fruits, milk, and meat and beans.

MyPyramid 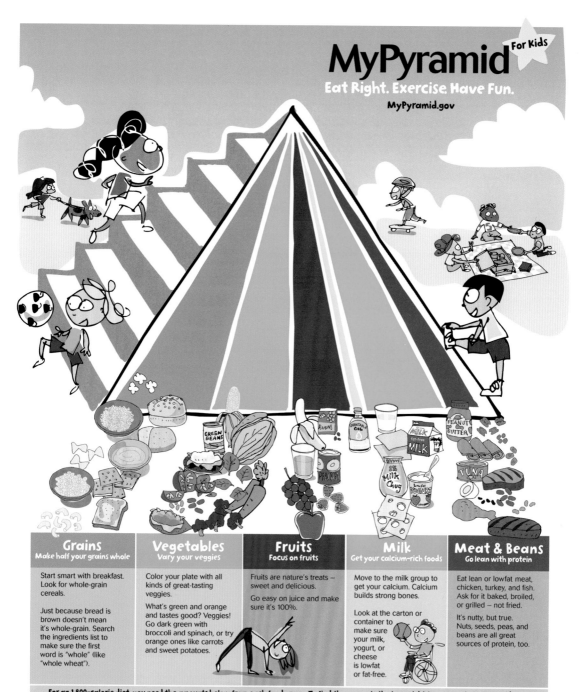 For Kids

Eat Right. Exercise Have Fun.

MyPyramid.gov

Grains	Vegetables	Fruits	Milk	Meat & Beans
Make half your grains whole	**Vary your veggies**	**Focus on fruits**	**Get your calcium-rich foods**	**Go lean with protein**
Start smart with breakfast. Look for whole-grain cereals. Just because bread is brown doesn't mean it's whole-grain. Search the ingredients list to make sure the first word is "whole" (like "whole wheat").	Color your plate with all kinds of great-tasting veggies. What's green and orange and tastes good? Veggies! Go dark green with broccoli and spinach, or try orange ones like carrots and sweet potatoes.	Fruits are nature's treats — sweet and delicious. Go easy on juice and make sure it's 100%.	Move to the milk group to get your calcium. Calcium builds strong bones. Look at the carton or container to make sure your milk, yogurt, or cheese is lowfat or fat-free.	Eat lean or lowfat meat, chicken, turkey, and fish. Ask for it baked, broiled, or grilled – not fried. It's nutty, but true. Nuts, seeds, peas, and beans are all great sources of protein, too.

For an 1,800-calorie diet, you need the amounts below from each food group. To find the amounts that are right for you, go to MyPyramid.gov.

Eat 6 oz. every day; at least half should be whole	Eat 2 ½ cups every day	Eat 1 ½ cups every day	Get 3 cups every day; for kids ages 2 to 8, it's 2 cups	Eat 5 oz. every day

Oils Oils are not a food group, but you need some for good health. Get your oils from fish, nuts, and liquid oils such as corn oil, soybean oil, and canola oil.

Find your balance between food and fun

- Move more. Aim for at least 60 minutes everyday, or most days.
- Walk, dance, bike, rollerblade – it all counts. How great is that!

Fats and sugars — know your limits

- Get your fat facts and sugar smarts from the Nutrition Facts label.
- Limit solid fats as well as foods that contain them.
- Choose food and beverages low in added sugars and other caloric sweeteners.

MyPyramid.gov
STEPS TO A HEALTHIER YOU

U.S. Department of Agriculture
Food and Nutrition Service
September 2005
FNS-381

CALORIES AT WORK			
Activity (1 Hour)	130 lbs.	155 lbs.	190 lbs.
Aerobics (moderate impact)	354	422	518
Backpacking (general)	413	493	604
Badminton (social)	266	317	388
Basketball (game)	472	563	690
Bicycling (leisure, <10 mph)	236	281	345
Bicycling (stationary, moderate effort)	413	493	604
Billiards	148	176	216
Bowling	177	211	259
Circuit Training	472	563	690
Construction (outdoor)	325	387	474
Cooking	148	176	216
Flag Football	472	563	690
Football (competitive)	531	633	776
Frisbee (ultimate)	207	246	302
Golf (carrying clubs)	325	387	474
Golf (miniature)	177	211	259
Hiking (cross-country)	354	422	518
Hockey (ice or field)	472	563	690
Jogging (general)	413	493	604
Jumping Rope (moderate)	590	704	863
Kick-boxing/Karate/Judo	590	704	863
Lacrosse	472	563	690
Mowing the lawn (push mower)	325	387	474
Running (ten-minute mile)	590	704	863
Skateboarding	295	352	431
Skiing (x-country, moderate effort)	472	563	690
Skiing (downhill, moderate effort)	354	422	518
Soccer (competitive)	590	704	863
Softball or baseball (fast or slow pitch)	295	352	431
Volleyball (picnic, 6-9 members team)	177	211	259
Walking the dog (moderate pace)	207	246	302
Walking (briskly – 4 m.p.h.)	236	281	345

CALORIES AND NUTRITION

All foods have calories, whether it's cookies or carrots, lettuce or ice cream, but some foods have more calories than others. This means that if you ate a pound of lettuce, you would have eaten only about 80 calories (and you would have had to eat about 16 cups of lettuce)—but if you ate a pound of chocolate chip cookies (about 10 cookies), you would have eaten 2,100 calories! That's a big difference.

Every day, your body needs *nutrition* from many kinds of foods. Different kinds of food contain different *nutrients*, and you need a balanced diet of all of them. Your body needs carbohydrates, fats, protein, and minerals and vitamins every day. The only way to get all you need of these nutrients is to eat lots of different kinds of healthy foods.

Nutrition is the process by which your body gets from food what it needs to be healthy. **Nutrients** are the things in food that help your body live and grow.

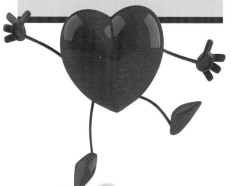

GET ACTIVE!

MyPyramid also shows you that your body not only needs you to eat right to be healthy—your body also needs you to move around and exercise. Your body was made to move. Your muscles are designed to pull your bones and bend your joints.

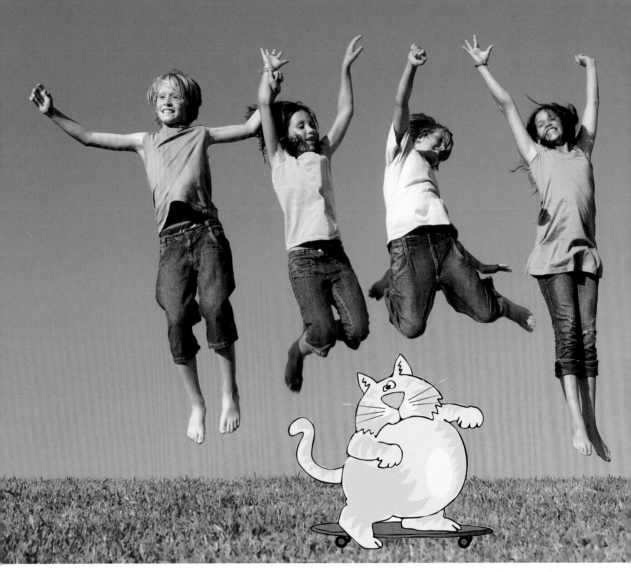

You don't have to play a sport to exercise—just jumping around and having fun is good for your body.

Nowadays, with people spending so much of their time sitting, it's hard to get the exercise we need.

When you exercise regularly, though, you not only help your body use calories in a healthy way, you also make all the cells and organs in your body healthier. When you're strong and fit, your body makes good use of the food you eat, and all your body parts are much more likely to work together the way they should. This means that even when you're not exercising, you use more calories. You feel better, physically and emotionally—and you even think better!

Sports are a great way to get the exercise you need, but even if you don't like sports, you can still keep your body healthy by running around and being active in lots of different ways.

The chart below gives you tips for how to eat right, exercise, stay healthy—and have fun!

TIPS FOR FAMILIES

EAT RIGHT

1 **Make half your grains whole.** Choose whole-grain foods, such as whole-wheat bread, oatmeal, brown rice, and lowfat popcorn, more often.

2 **Vary your veggies.** Go dark green and orange with your vegetables—eat spinach, broccoli, carrots, and sweet potatoes.

3 **Focus on fruits.** Eat them at meals, and at snack time, too. Choose fresh, frozen, canned, or dried, and go easy on the fruit juice.

4 **Get your calcium-rich foods.** To build strong bones serve lowfat and fat-free milk and other milk products several times a day.

5 **Go lean with protein.** Eat lean or lowfat meat, chicken, turkey, and fish. Also, change your tune with more dry beans and peas. Add chick peas, nuts, or seeds to a salad; pinto beans to a burrito; or kidney beans to soup.

6 **Change your oil.** We all need oil. Get yours from fish, nuts, and liquid oils such as corn, soybean, canola, and olive oil.

7 **Don't sugarcoat it.** Choose foods and beverages that do not have sugar and caloric sweeteners as one of the first ingredients. Added sugars contribute calories with few, if any, nutrients.

EXERCISE

1 **Set a good example.** Be active and get your family to join you. Have fun together. Play with the kids or pets. Go for a walk, tumble in the leaves, or play catch.

2 **Take the President's Challenge as a family.** Track your individual physical activities together and earn awards for active lifestyles at *www.presidentschallenge.org*.

3 **Establish a routine.** Set aside time each day as activity time—walk, jog, skate, cycle, or swim. Adults need at least 30 minutes of physical activity most days of the week; children 60 minutes everyday or most days.

4 **Have an activity party.** Make the next birthday party centered on physical activity. Try backyard Olympics, or relay races. Have a bowling or skating party.

5 **Set up a home gym.** Use household items, such as canned foods, as weights. Stairs can substitute for stair machines.

6 **Move it!** Instead of sitting through TV commercials, get up and move. When you talk on the phone, lift weights or walk around. Remember to limit TV watching and computer time.

7 **Give activity gifts.** Give gifts that encourage physical activity—active games or sporting equipment.

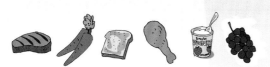

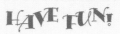
HAVE FUN!

CHAPTER

4 WHY DOES IT MATTER?

Eating is fun. And maybe YOU don't have a weight problem. Or maybe you do, but you really don't care. After all, being overweight doesn't mean you aren't also smart and funny and good looking. It doesn't mean people don't like you, and it certainly does NOT mean you should feel bad about yourself. No matter how much you weigh, whether you're skinny or heavy or somewhere in the middle, you're an amazing and special person. You have gifts to give the world that only you can give!

And because that's true, because you ARE so special, you need to take care of yourself. You need to do everything you can to be sure you stay healthy.

FICTION

FACT

Lots of health problems can come from being overweight or obese. If you weigh too much, the extra weight can damage your joints. It can change the way you breathe and sleep, and it can also change your moods, and energy levels. Your entire life can be changed by being overweight.

That's why you need to think about what you eat. Don't make the mistake of thinking that bigger is always better!

HEALTHY WEIGHT EQUALS HEALTHY BODIES

Children who are overweight or obese are more likely to get diabetes. This is a disease where your body doesn't break down sugar the way it should. If you have diabetes, you will probably have to take medicine or have special shots every day to help your body process sugar. Diabetes can lead to other diseases as well, including blindness. It can make it hard for you to heal after a cut or injury.

When you see an enormous hamburger it may look amazing and wonderful to you—but remember that healthy eating means eating smaller portions.

Being overweight also increases your chances of having heart disease. This is an illness we usually connect with older people, but carrying too much weight around is hard on your heart, no matter how old you are. Even worse, the heavier you are, the harder it will probably be for you to run around and exercise. Your heart and lungs need exercise to be healthy. Today, more and more children are obese or overweight—and more and more children are getting heart disease.

Overweight children are also likely to stay that way as they grow up. Being obese or overweight when you are an adult can put you at risk for even more diseases. Obesity may even cause certain kinds of *cancer*.

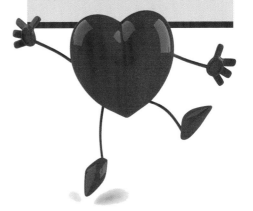

Cancer is a disease that causes some cells in your body to grow too fast, to the point that they kill healthy, normal cells.

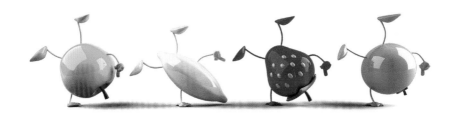

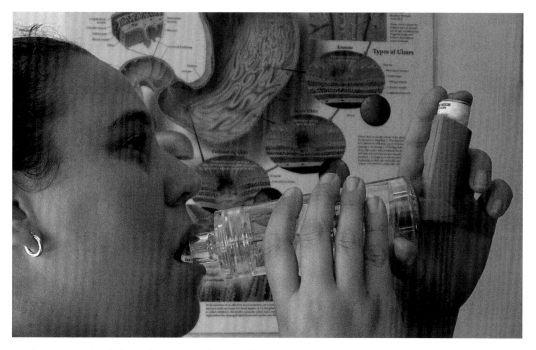

Children and adults who are overweight are more likely to have asthma, which makes it difficult for them to breathe normally.

DID YOU KNOW?

At least 2.6 million people each year die as a result of being overweight or obese.

As people who are overweight or obese grow older, the added weight on their bodies can also lead to other problems, like high blood pressure (which increases your chances of having a stroke), and breathing problems. Being overweight can also mean that you have more problems handling your emotions. People who are obese or over-weight are often more likely to feel sad.

SO WHAT SHOULD YOU DO?

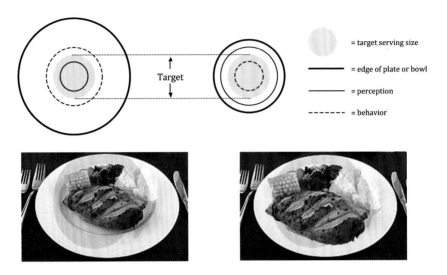

Even though you're still a kid, there are things you can do to make sure you take care of yourself by eating in a way that's good for you, that won't make you gain weight as you get older. Pay attention to how big your food portions are. Talk to

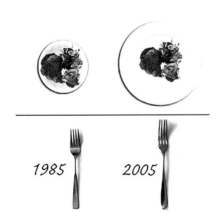

1985   2005

your parents and the other adults in your life about how you can all choose better serving sizes. Use smaller plates to help you eat less. (See the chart at the top of this page.) Learn what a serving looks like by reading the chart on the next page.

Portion Size Guidelines

Below are ways you can picture a serving or portion size using everyday objects. *(Note: hands and finger sizes vary from person to person! These are **GUIDES** only).*

Food Portion   ## Looks Like

Grains, Beans, and Starchy Vegetables Group

½ cup cooked rice or pasta.................................**half of a baseball**

½ cup cooked dry beans, lentils, or peas ....cupcake wrapper full

½ cup potatoes, corn, green peas ....level ice cream scoop

corn on the cob ....4-inch corn cob

Vegetable

1 cup green salad ....baseball or a fist

¾ cup tomato juice...small styrofoam cup

½ cup cooked broccoli ....half baseball or **light bulb**

½ cup serving ....6 asparagus spears,
7 or 8 baby carrots

Fruit

½ cup of fresh fruit ....custard cup

1 medium size fruit...**fist** or baseball

¼ cup raisins...large egg

The Meat and Protein Foods

3 ounces cooked meat, fish, poultry ....**deck of cards**

3 ounces cooked chicken....................................leg plus thigh or ½ whole breast

1 ounce of cheese ....4 stacked dice

2 tablespoons peanut butter ....ping-pong ball

1 teaspoon peanut butter....................................fingertip

1 tablespoon peanut butter ....**thumb tip**

Fats, Oils and Nuts

1 teaspoon butter, margarine..............................**fingertip**

2 tablespoons salad dressing ....ping-pong ball

Did you to know that...

- **1 cupped hand** holds 2 tablespoons of liquid.
- 1 slice of bread is one ounce or 1 serving;
some rolls or bagels weigh 3 to 5 ounces or more
making them equal to 3 to 5 servings of bread

Missouri Department of Health & Senior Services
Bureau of Cancer and Chronic Disease Control

ENJOY YOUR FOOD

Eating less doesn't mean you have to stop liking food. It doesn't mean you have to feel empty and hungry all the time.

In fact, if you take time to think about what you're eating, you may find you enjoy it more. Don't just shovel as much food into your mouth as you can in as short a time possible!

Instead, make meals special times where you enjoy being with the people you like. Make the table look nice. Arrange the dishes and put flowers on the table. Talk about interesting things. *Celebrate* the happy feelings of being together.

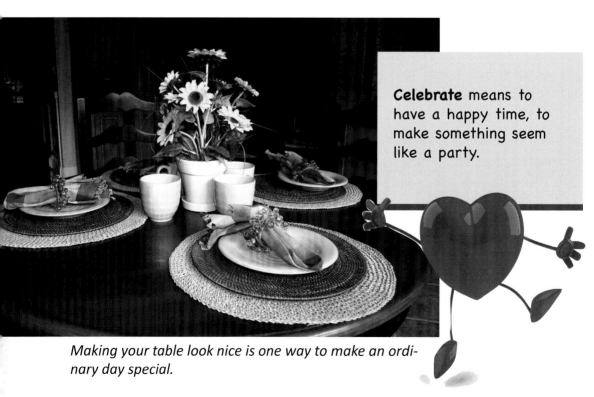

Celebrate means to have a happy time, to make something seem like a party.

Making your table look nice is one way to make an ordinary day special.

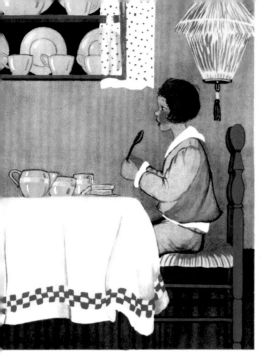

Even if you're eating alone, think about the tastes of the foods you're eating. Pay attention to the different flavors. Notice the way the food feels in your mouth.

Eating SHOULD be fun!

You may find it's easier to eat less if you think about enjoying the people you're with while you eat.

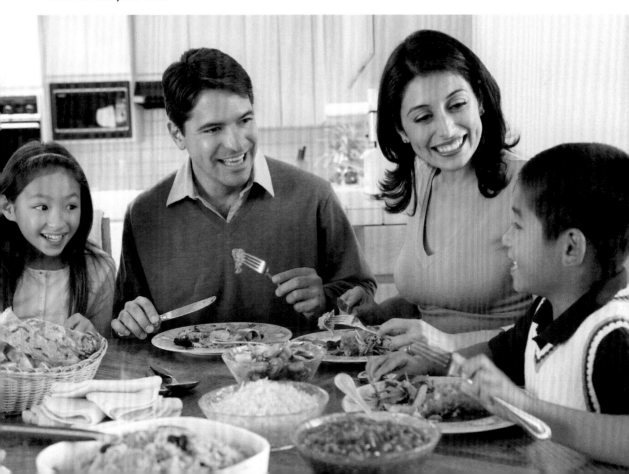

SLOW DOWN, EAT LESS

Our world seems to be always in a hurry. But you can choose to slow down.

Instead of eating fast food, make a new habit—eat slow. Take your time when you eat. Chew your food carefully. Don't gulp it down. Don't rush. You'll find you'll eat less when you eat slowly.

BE A PICKY EATER!

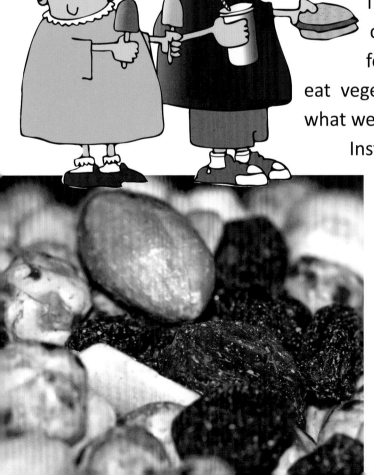

Maybe your mom and dad scold you sometimes for being a picky eater. They probably mean you don't like to try new foods, or you don't like to eat vegetables. And that's NOT what we mean here.

Instead, we mean you should learn to pick the foods that are healthiest. Whole or unprocessed foods—in other words, foods that are as close as possible to the way they grew naturally, without being fro-

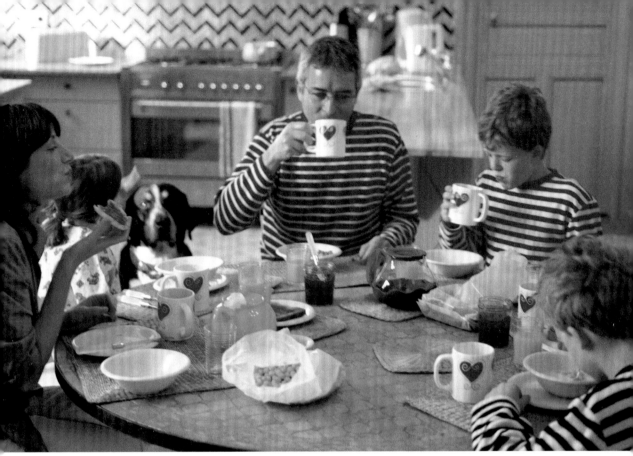

Meal times shouldn't be rushed. They should be chances for people to enjoy being with each other while they catch up on each other's lives.

zen, canned, or packaged—are the best choices for getting what your body needs.

Does this mean you have to give up foods like potato chips, candy bars, and cookies forever? No, it's okay to have these foods once in a while. Just don't eat too many of them. To choose healthier foods, check food labels, and then pick foods that are high in vitamins and minerals.

That's the RIGHT kind of picky eater, the kind who remembers that bigger isn't always better!

READ MORE ABOUT IT

Bean, Anita. *Awesome Foods for Active Kids: The ABCs of Eating for Energy and Health.* Alameda, Calif.: Hunter House, 2006.

Behan, Eileen. *Fit Kids: Raising Physically and Emotionally Strong Kids with Real Food.* New York: Pocket Publishing, 2001.

Dolgoff, Joanna. *Red Light, Green Light, Eat Right: The Food Solution That Lets Kids Be Kids.* Emmaus, Penn.: Rodale, 2009.

Zinczenko, David and Matt Goulding. *Eat This Not That! For Kids!* Emmaus, Penn.: Rodale, 2008.

FIND OUT MORE ON THE INTERNET

Move It!
www.fns.usda.gov/tn/tnrockyrun/moveit.htm

MyPyramid Blast Off Game
www.mypyramid.gov/kids/kids_game.html

Small Step Kids
www.smallstep.gov/kids/html/games_and_activities.html

INDEX

ABOUT THE AUTHOR

Rae Simons has ghostwritten several adult books on dieting and obesity. She is also the author of more than thirty young adult books. She lives in upstate New York, where she tries hard to get enough exercise and eat healthy foods.

PICTURE CREDITS